"SNATCHES
AN EXPLANATORY
EPI

BY
PEGGY HUME

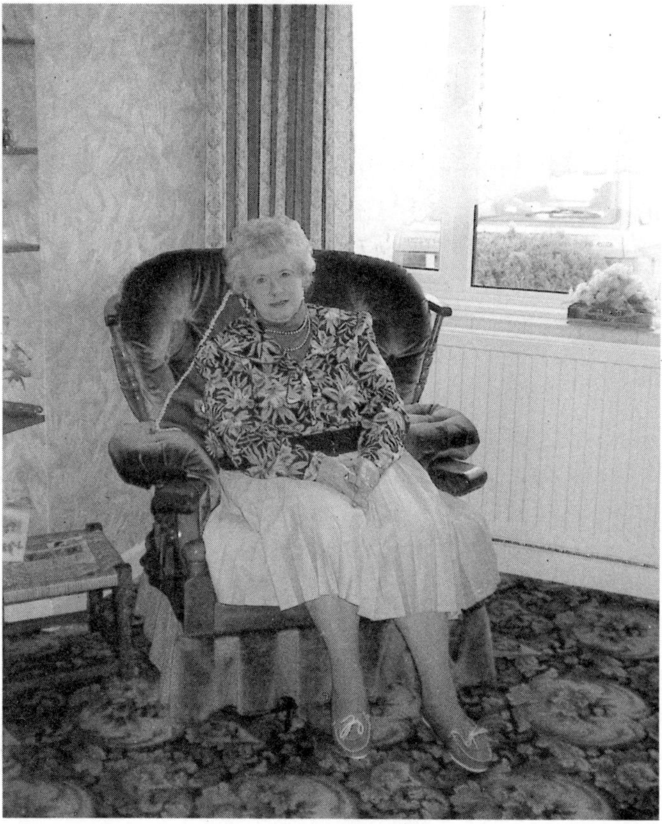

Copyright © 2003 Peggy Hume

All rights reserved. No part of this publication may be reproduced, stored in a retrieval system, or transmitted in any form by means, electronic, mechanical, photocopying, recording or otherwise, without the prior permission of the copyright owner.

First published in the United Kingdom in 2003 by:
PEGGY HUME
39a, Theatre Street,
Woodbridge
Suffolk IP12 4NE

A CIP catalogue record is available for this book from the
British Library
ISBN 0 9546519-0-1

Printed & bound in Great Britain by:
Bettaprint, 1 Carlow Mews, Church Street, Woodbridge, Suffolk IP12 1EA

"Snatches of Living"
by
Peggy Hume

Contents.

Section		Page
1	Introduction	5
2	Types of Epilepsy	8
3	When, How & Why?	12
4	Diagnosis	14
5	Tests	15
6	Treatment & Trials	18
7	Drugs	21
8	Disadvantages of being an Epileptic	24
9	Disadvantages Healthwise	26
10	Accidents caused by Epilepsy	28
11	Identification	31
12	Hobbies and Interests	32

****

Chapters

1	"Snatches of living", my life	35
2	10yrs to 14yrs	38
3	Teenage Years	43
4	Work	46
5	Teenage Romances	49
6	Marriage and Children	52
7	Where is Home?	58
8	Planning the rest of my life - Travel	60
9	Cairo	64
10	Back home in England	65
11	A True Friend	67
12	Summary of life as an Epileptic	71

ACKNOWLEDGEMENT

As the author of this book, I wish to thank Mark and James of Bettaprint Printers at Woodbridge in Suffolk for their patience & help in enabling me to get this book out on time.

Thank you.

Section 1

INTRODUCTION

There are in Gt Britain an average 500,000 registered Epileptics. There are probably many more who are not registered. People who have developed some form of Epilepsy, but feel themselves very embarrassed admitting to others that they suffer from the brain disorder, regardless of whichever form they suffer from. It is just not something you talk about to others. I am sure that many sufferers will be able to identify with me concerning many of the problems and encounters of which I shall speak throughout this book.

I have given my book the title "Snatches of Living" as that is exactly what my life was until recently. When younger I would often only just recover from one seizure and a few hours later I had another, so about half of my life has been spent in bed sleeping off many of the seizures which have occurred throughout over sixty years of my life.

People's understanding of Epilepsy and awareness of the problems sufferers can come up against are rarely mentioned. If I had Cancer or some other serious disease then everyone would feel sorry for me and help in any way they could to ease the burden of my illness, but with Epilepsy, generally people do not to want to get involved.

I do not intend this to be a 'heavy' medical journal, although I have given the main details necessary to understand Epilepsy and how and why it happens. I am writing this for families, friends and associates of Epileptics mainly (medical teams may also learn something from it), in the hope that they can better understand the sufferer's feelings at the time of a seizure, after and other instances.

I have covered incidents right from the first days of being an epileptic as a five year old child through teens, work, marriage, children, social life right up to the present time of being an over sixty year old pensioner. Life has presented many different types of problems through each of these stages of my life. These I have covered.

I would like to point out here, that although I have suffered from Epilepsy all my life and all my experiences are true, I am NOT a doctor and if you are troubled in any way with ill health then I must recommend that you speak to your GP.

My final reason for writing this book, is that sitting in the living-room at a computer is safer than crossing the road when you are an epileptic!

* * * * * * * * * *

Part 1

Section 2

TYPES OF EPILEPSY

There are many different types of Epilepsy but I think the three most habitual are Grand Mal now known as Tonic Clonic, then the Petit Mal now known as Absence Seizure and Nocturnal Epilepsy. Why they have now changed these names is very confusing for one of us older epilepsy sufferers. I myself throughout my life have been unfortunate enough to suffer from all three of these forms of epilepsy which I shall refer to by the name I have always known them by.

GRAND MAL EPILEPSY : Has in my case been the most severe form of Epilepsy. When a seizure takes place the victim of this disease usually appears to others to have a blank face with staring eyes, they then usually scream out. The body stiffens then jerks spasmodically. In these few seconds one often bites the tongue and the inside of the mouth; this can be very painful for the person having the seizure. These injuries can take weeks to heal and are not very pleasant to live with, as I know to my cost.

There are many other more serious injuries which can occur whilst having a seizure; they can even induce a heart attack or stroke. I know, I have spent much of my life recovering from injuries incurred during having seizures. But having said that, I have always recovered from the attacks eventually and got on with my life.

Whilst on the subject of recovering, there is a misconception that once the eyes open an epileptic is fully conscious immediately. Very rarely is this so. Usually when a person comes round from an epileptic seizure it takes the brain at least 30 minutes, sometimes longer, after waking up to read just to normal thinking. The brain definitely does NOT return to normal straight away. The brain cells which were scrambled in the seizure by an electrical storm need time to settle down properly once again.

This one subject makes me angry when films and TV documentaries are made about epileptics, often where the sufferer jumps up on waking and starts conversing and doing whatever they were doing before the seizure occurred. Epilepsy does not work like that.
After seeing these happenings as I have described on films and documentaries I have written/phoned the film makers and asked where they got their information regarding the subject of epilepsy. Usually their answer is The Epilepsy Society. I have then phoned the Epilepsy Societies and asked if all their staff were epileptics, of course the answer was NO. So there you have it, unless you are an epileptic how can you know exactly how an epileptic feels on coming round from a seizure; even doctors don't know that!

If only these film makers could ask us EPILEPTICS the necessary: How/Why/Where/When. We are the only ones who really know how it feels being an epileptic and coming around from a seizure. If these facts are not given correctly then all people will have the wrong information about epilepsy and how to treat sufferers. We are human we just have a brain disorder which we cannot control. That's all.

GRAND MAL : People witnessing a person having a Grand Mal seizure often at this stage attempt to push things in the mouth; hankies, spoons etc but this action is a waste of time because the victim has by then bitten their tongue, if they are going to.

After the seizure is too late. I can appreciate that these people are well-meaning but it does not help and I can assure you it is not a very pleasant experience to have any of these objects rammed into your mouth when you are trying to recover from the seizure. The blinding headaches I have always been left with are not very pleasant either. Bed and sleep is usually the best thing after these types of seizures, often for four or five hours sleep and everything is back to normal. Apart from a very bad migraine type of headache.

PETIT MAL EPILEPSY : Now called an Absence Seizure. This type of Epilepsy can start at any time in life; as can the others. I have also had these periodically for all my life. I will just say that the effects of this type of epilepsy rarely leaves me with the headache like the Grand Mal does. I just have this blank 'strange' feeling and if one is talking to me I do not hear what they are saying for a few minutes. The after effects of this type of epilepsy are much easier to cope with, (although at times when with someone it can be embarrassing). Sometimes I just feel a bit dopey for about five or ten minutes and then I am all right again.

If I had to make a choice, this would be the type of Epilepsy I would settle for.... But what a choice to have to make! At least Petit Mal seizures are much less humiliating as the victim is not usually caught in the compromising positions which can occur with Grand Mal seizures.

NOCTURNAL EPILEPSY : As the name states, this form of epilepsy occurs whilst the patient is in bed sleeping. I had this form of epilepsy very bad when I was young; My body would start shaking and jerking whilst I was sleeping; very often I would end up falling out of the bed from the jerking around the bed. When I was a child Mum would come in to me and settle me back in bed. She had as many sleepless nights as I had! After the seizure had gone I would go back to sleep only to awake the next morning with a blinding headache...a very bad start to the day when I went to work.

This form of epilepsy continued regularly until I was about 35 years old but now it does not happen so often, but it does happen sometimes.

There are, apparently other forms of epilepsy. I have not had them so I cannot comment on them as I am not one of them or a doctor, just a victim of the three types mentioned. On the subject of doctors, most of them are quite sympathetic, but even they; unless they are also sufferers, can have no idea of what it is like to live with epilepsy. The Neurologists I have seen have been very helpful, but they are still not the sufferers. Epilepsy is a cruel complaint over which you have no control at all. IT never warns you when IT is about to strike you down and turn your world upside down as it often can. IT alienates you, the sufferer from so many people. Most people, although not all, choose to keep away from you, not because of the person you are when you are alright but not wanting, or being afraid of the responsibility which epilepsy may bring. If epilepsy was talked about more then probably these attitudes would disappear but the subject is taboo. Don't mention it.

These attitudes can be very hurtful, we can't help being epileptic, it certainly is not an illness we chose to have! So us sufferers spend most of our years with epilepsy trying to prove to others that, when we are 'standing' we are just as capable as any other person. Sadly not many people accept this. But some do.

Section 3

WHEN, HOW AND WHY?

Epilepsy usually starts in childhood, before the age of eighteen. There are, of course exceptions; especially if the person has had an accident or suffered head injuries of some kind. Drug abuse and alcohol can also start epilepsy. Having said that it can also start when people get older, especially after a stroke. There is no definite time really for epilepsy to start or finish. Your brain alone will make that decision.

In children the epilepsy usually starts very young, but by the time they reach eighteen it can cease completely. This is not to say that it will not return at a later date; no-one can ever say for certain. I have spent my life praying for them not to come back. Epilepsy is the sort of brain disorder that can lie dormant for many years before showing itself again. No one can ever be sure that it will not re-occur.

One person in about every two-hundred will, at some time in their life experience the torment of epilepsy. It may seem so mild that you cannot diagnose it. This often happens when the person fails to seek help from a doctor. Of course it may turn out to be just short-term but it may be permanent. No-one can tell. It is not as rare as some think.

HOW DOES EPILEPSY HAPPEN? : As I understand it the brain is made up of millions of nerve cells called neurones all connected to each other. These travel constantly through our brain telling our brain and body how to act. Their job is to organize messages which it receives. When the messages are no longer required, then in a healthy person the brain will cancel out the messages not required anymore. In Epilepsy, however, the sufferers brain often fails to do this job properly, this induces electrical charges in the brain by the overloading and a seizure takes place. Epilepsy often occurs in people who are brainy. But the brain when it works overtime, overloads itself. That's when a seizure takes place. So Epilepsy, in its own way is really a safety release plus it warns the sufferer to slow down from work, study or excitement; whatever is overloading their brain. The trouble is it doesn't usually stop us for long. I have told myself very sternly to slow down, but once we get interested in something again or are enjoying ourselves we tend to forget what the consequences can be...a seizure.

IS EPILEPSY INHERITED? : Apparently not directly, but a child in any family where epilepsy has occurred (not necessarily the next generation) can inherit a low seizure threshold against epilepsy from one parent. This can induce epilepsy itself but usually the other parent, having a higher threshold against epilepsy will ward of any attacks. Should both parents have a high threshold against epilepsy then it is highly unlikely that any children of these parents will contract any form of epilepsy; unless of course one has an unfortunate accident which can damage the brain. This, however, is nothing to do with hereditary forms of epilepsy. So it is not the epilepsy which is inherited but the genetic make-up for or against the development of epilepsy.

My own second daughter has never had children. This is probably because she abhors the thought that the child might be an epileptic. This was, I think the best decision because she certainly never, ever showed me any sympathy when I had seizures in front of her. I got the impression over the years that, to her, I was an embarrassment, but as I have said before, epilepsy is not an ailment anyone chooses to have to live with. It just happens and the victim has no control over when and where it will happen.

My son, on the other hand was always there to help me and much more caring and sympathetic towards my being epileptic. He now has a daughter of his own. It just depends on the person I suppose. But we never, any of us, know what is around the corner do we? So how can we judge others.

Section 4

DIAGNOSIS

When epilepsy is first diagnosed by your G.P or the hospital, relying on the information which you provide him with, he will then probably prescribe for you some anti-epileptic drug. In some cases this action is all it takes to control the seizures. In other cases, however, as with myself then the seizures may still continue; some drugs can make them worse. If this happens then the doctor will usually then arrange for you to see a neurologist at the hospital and do tests.

In many cases, however, increased amounts of drugs do not always work, If that brand which you are prescribed does not work for you then others will be tried so do not give up hope. I myself, over the years tried many different anti-epileptic drugs and only now at over sixty have I come up with the most reliable; Tegretol (Carbamazepine) are the ones I take and they work well for me. They have not completely stopped the seizures, but they have helped enormously in controlling the amount of seizures I have. One has to be grateful for small mercies.

I can go four to six months now between seizures but that can be cut shorter or longer depending on my life style at the time. The more hectic my life, i.e. worries, excitement etc then the more likely I am to have a seizure. Most things which get the brain working overtime can induce a seizure if you are an epileptic. For instance, when I had the children and was married the perplexities of married life and a violent husband, made my epilepsy very bad; three seizures a day sometimes. But now these worries have been removed from my life and I live a much calmer lifestyle the epileptic seizures have also decreased; with the help of these tablets. I just wish that they would disappear completely. Maybe one day.

Section 5

TESTS

It is very difficult nowadays to get an appointment with a neurologist immediately; most waiting lists are about 4-6 months. This can cause a lot of frustration for the victim of the epilepsy, neither knowing definitely what is wrong or how it can be cured. I can sympathise with anyone in this predicament especially if the seizures take over your life as they did mine.

I went from hospital to hospital in the 1950's and 60's seeing many different surgeons. I even went as far afield from my home in Suffolk to St James Square, in London. They asked questions such as.... Did I smoke? Did I drink? Did I take other drugs? I was desperate and impatient at this time for the seizures to stop. I was married with three children & a husband and had already endured 20 yrs of Epileptic seizures. I could see no relevance in these questions at the time with me having seizures, I just wanted them to stop.

The epilepsy, when I was 25 yrs old was still occurring roughly twice every day. I co-operated fully during these tests, in the hope that out of these interviews and tests something good would happen; like the banishing of the seizures. What a dream.

I was living with a constant headache and trying to bring up three children under five years of age. The day of the tests I was not even sure I was going to make it on the train back to Woodbridge, in Suffolk after all this stress! What you have to remember is that 50 years ago when I first had these tests the technology was not as advanced as it is now. Now they can detect almost any abnormality.

I had blood tests first, then the EEG or Electroencephalogram as I think is the technical term. This was a machine that recorded my brain wave activities. The problem here is that this test could only record the patterns for that particular day in question, so if you were feeling reasonably well that particular day, with no worries then the irregularities of the brain would probably not show up.

That day at Queen's Square, London seemed quite frightening to me. I sat in a large chair with lots of electrodes pressed onto my scalp. They apparently record the brainwaves at the time of the test. Sitting in that chair reminded me of someone going to the Electric Chair to die, same principle, just not quite as final I hoped. I tried to free my mind of that scary feeling. The brain, apparently needed to be free for the tests they told me.

Next, more tests were done where they shone flashing lights at me. I reacted strongly to these. I have always had the same sensitive reaction to strong lights: When I was younger in dance halls, and worst of all whilst sitting relaxed at home and watching Television. NOW, there are, on our televisions so many advertisements with thousands of flashing lights. I know they want our attention but do they never think that literally millions of people hate this, especially epileptics. I wish the makers of these ads would have a little sympathy for many of us epileptics...things like this can induce an epileptic seizure!

After all these days tests, I was thanked for my co-operation and told that was all and they would be in touch with my doctor at a later date...they never gave me any indication of what was going on, what was wrong or anything. This action upset me as it is my body and brain and I wanted to know what was going on and how to put it right. Hospitals are more helpful now in the 2000's than they were in the 1950's.

A few weeks later the doctors decided to try me on Phenytoin (Epanutin) but these never worked for me. They actually increased the seizures as did Primidone (Mysoline) which they tried next.

But trying to be a good enduring patient I stuck it out for the next four years - what a waste of my life - and then I complained strongly to my doctor. Then I was put on a stronger dose of Phenobarbitone again plus Garoin.

I spent the next TEN YEARS walking around in a dream, like a zombie, full of anti-epileptic drugs, but still having at least one seizure a day. By this time I had had enough, my life was being wasted by spending a third of every day sleeping off seizures. This is where I got the title for this book "Snatches of Living".

I went back to my doctor demanding someone to help me. I had had enough. I had wasted 45 years being an epileptic, I wanted to live a little, soon it would be too late to appreciate living! Just a few hours/days/ years free of seizures, if possible.

* * * * * * * * * *

Section 6

TREATMENT AND TRIALS

The next set of tests took place in 1984 at Ipswich Hospital. I was by then 49yrs old. I had an MRI scan, which I was told was better than the EEG. It entailed, once more, having lots of metal plates stuck to my head. I was laid flat on my back on a bed. The bed slid slowly into a low tunnel. As I suffer slightly from claustrophobia the tests were done in short ten -minute sessions. A very frightening experience, but I would have done anything to be free of these Epileptic seizures.

The MRI took pictures of my brain; they were now more advanced in technology than in the 1950's and 1960's. It was later assessed that one of the problems was that the Temporal Lobe area of my brain was damaged and causing the epilepsy. So armed with this brief piece of information I went home and waited for the hospital consultant's decision on the appropriate treatment for the future.

About a month later I was once more summoned to the hospital and told of the decision to change my tablets to help control the seizures. To do this I had to be admitted into hospital for one month to drain my body completely of any other anti-epileptic drugs before starting these new ones; a combination of Tegretol and Epilim supposedly a good combination. I was willing to try anything; I had endured Epilepsy long enough.

* * * * * * * * * * *

This next period in hospital was terrifying for me. I was not given any medication for epilepsy but drained completely of anti-epileptic drugs. Whilst this was happening; about two weeks, I was having seizures constantly. They put me in a side ward and strapped me down for safety. Once the body was cleansed of drugs they gradually introduced the Tegretol and Epilim. Now the real test was about to take place. Would they work? Maybe, I wanted them to.

After about a week the seizures had declined slightly but not as much as the neurologist had hoped. He then withdrew the Epilim and continued with the Tegretol. From then on things improved and the seizures lessened, I sometimes went days without a seizure. After about a month in hospital I went home and the seizures were definitely less frequent. But they still, to this day, have not gone completely as I wish they would. I can, if lucky, go three-four months now without a seizure, but I can never be sure how long I will go because epilepsy is, as I said, very unpredictable. But life is certainly better than it was fifteen years ago when I was having two to three seizures a day.

There are now operations which can be performed on the brain to repair the cause of the Epilepsy which is wonderful progress; I just wish they would repair mine. The brain is a very serious part to tamper with and it must be a very difficult operation but to my mind as an epileptic sufferer, it would be worth it. Lets be honest, what good is it having to spend at least a third of your life being laid out on the floor unconscious when, if you had an operation, you could have a ninety per cent chance or more of being cured. It can work as I have both read about and seen on television. I know I would take the chance if it were offered to me.

Epilepsy restricts the sufferers' quality of life very strongly. The 'normal' person spends about a third of their life sleeping. Being epileptic can increase that to two thirds or more, recovering from seizures. Silly little things which people take for granted like having an argument, getting excited, worrying, these ordinary everyday activities are the very things which can cause an epileptic to have a seizure.

My life has been a continuous fight with my brain to try to overcome Epilepsy. Twenty years ago I was advised to try meditation classes. I was very sceptical but I tried them and it calmed me a bit, but I am not going to say that it stopped me having seizures because it never had that positive an action it just slowed my brain down for the odd fifteen minutes.

* * * * * * * * * *

Section 7

<u>DRUGS</u>

There are now many good Anti-Epileptic drugs on the market. Research has advanced in this field. The ones I have used are: Epilim, Phenobarbitone, Phenytoin, Mysoline and Tegretol which I am using now. There are, of course others but I, not being a doctor have no knowledge of them myself. Your own doctor can help you there.

Some of these drugs can leave you with a very drowsy, dopey feeling because of the strength you may be considered to need. They can leave you fighting with your brain and body to do something with your life, but the drug takes over and slows down your brain; they are supposed to do that. This in turn makes it very difficult to concentrate even on reading a book...a very simple task to someone who is not plagued with Epilepsy.

This may all sound very boring; that one has to take this medication everyday without fail but if you wish to be free even for one day of epileptic seizures then they really are necessary. It's a question of choice, not a very good one...If you take the tablets you may well be free of seizures at least for part of the time, if you don't take them then you will probably continue to have uncontrolled seizures. It really is your choice. I know which I would choose..the tablets definitely. I might add here that Epilepsy can induce heart attacks from which you could die, if not controlled.

DRUG TRIALS...It's simply a matter of being willing to try many different anti-epileptic drugs until you find which suits your brain best. I had forty-five years of trials to get to the tablets which suit me. These seem well suited to me but it has taken an immense amount of time and patience through all the trials and failings, but it was worth it in the end.

One point worth making here whilst on the subject of trying drugs is the misconception that just because the lady up the road takes one specific brand of tablets and they work for her that they will automatically work for you. It does not work like that, each person is an individual and must be treated as such.

I must have tried at least eight brands of tablets, probably many more, which I cannot recall, it's been a very frustrating sixty odd years, with all those trials and results shadowing my life. I have also had to take combinations of tablets, but that method never worked for me. When I had the Tegretol and Epilim I ended up more often on the floor having a seizure than before. But the Tegretol worked alone.

I have given in to the fact that my dream of escaping from the dreaded torment of being plagued with Epilepsy is probably never going to come true. The next best for me is at least to have a few days of freedom from them some of the time. Even being slowed down by drugs is, in a sense better than Epilepsy plus once the brain adjusts to the tablets the dopey feeling seems to lessen.

Whilst on the subject of tablets I would mention that people with Epilepsy, on medication, should NOT take the vitamins Folic Acid or Evening Primrose, apparently they fight with epilepsy medication. Some of the Antacids medicines which I have taken for indigestion have induced epileptic seizures; very violent ones. I doubt if anyone will believe me but peppermints, if taken near the time of taking the Tegretol can also starts my seizures sometimes. Apparently Tegretol have an ingredient in which also works on the digestion. I know this is true because after taking it I often get burping periods. I have now stopped eating peppermints, not because I wanted to and things are not quite so bad. Tegretol definitely 'fights' with numerous drugs, as I have found out to my peril. They want to be in charge, and they are!!

As I have already said, I am not a doctor, even though I have studied medicine at home. I always wanted to be a doctor but there again being an epileptic stopped that. But I have observed my own body and its reactions throughout life. Some I have found out the hard way, including the vitamins we all think are safe. They may be safe if you are NOT on medication for Epilepsy, but if you are, be cautious. Stimulants/ Vitamins like Omega 3 and others work against the job of the anti-epileptic drugs. Gen Sing is another fatal vitamin to take if you are epileptic and it makes sense because Epilepsy drugs SLOW YOU DOWN and vitamins like Gen Sing are to LIVEN YOU UP, so they fight in your body for supremacy. Believe me the Epilepsy drugs always win. I tried endless times to 'wake' the brain up and took all kinds of these vitamins but they work against epilepsy drugs and the consequences are a seizure. I gave up eventually when I realized just what was happening.

You can talk with your doctor about the effects of these combinations, some doctors don't even understand these vitamins and their reaction to real drugs, they don't have the time. But if we did mention our findings the doctor would probably think us patients were hypochondriacs! But definitely more research into these combinations should be done.

* * * * * * * * * *

Section 8

DISADVANTAGES OF BEING AN EPILEPTIC

You have to understand that an epileptic is constantly vulnerable. The instant the brain starts to work overtime, be it through worry, excitement, stress or whatever then that's usually the time the victim has a seizure. There is not a thing anyone can do to stop the seizure occurring.

All through life we will encounter numerous trials and tribulations, the kinds most people cope with quite easily. An Epileptic, however, does not have that privilege; the choice is taken over by the brain. My life has been a constant fight with my brain for the supremacy of making decisions for myself!

Epilepsy can have a major impact on your life, causing numerous problems throughout. Many aspects of life which most people find easy, are not so when you are an epileptic. The brain makes all your decisions for you. A stupid thing like crossing from one side of the road to the other on a pedestrian crossing can be a life threatening situation as I found out when I had a seizure on the pedestrian crossing in Oxford St in London! If a seizure happens at this moment then you are in trouble.

Social life can become nearly non-existent, ruled largely by epilepsy. The excitement and music can interfere with the brain. Drink does not help and there you are really enjoying yourself, loving life...its quite likely a seizure will occur at this very time when you really do not need it.

We, as epileptics have a real yearn to be normal, well I do anyway. To be able to do all the things which HEALTHY people take for granted every day of their lives. The victim of epilepsy can be one minute at a party happily engaged in talking and dancing and impressing some partner and then in a second can be laid out on the floor, shaking and screaming and even wetting oneself having an epileptic attack. Not a very pretty sight for someone who has never seen it happen before, and so terribly, terribly embarrassing for the victim. That's another crowd of people whom you will probably never, ever, see again. That I am sorry to say is how life goes on for the epileptic...from one crisis to another!

Epilepsy can cancel out all forms of romantic notions you may have for any person...well it probably will, once they see you having a seizure! Before that moment they will treat you the same as anyone else, but after seeing you having a seizure, often their attitude changes. Don't get me wrong, there are some people, who, after the event can actually sit down later and laugh with you about it. These gems of people, however, are very hard to find.

Another misconception I would like to correct is that an observer seeing an epileptic coming round from a seizure assumes that they are immediately in control of all their faculties and recognise the person who is speaking to them and remember where they are and feel fine. This is rarely true, well it never has been for me. Not with my Grand Mal seizures anyway. The patient can take up to at least thirty minutes to an hour to be reasonably in control once more. Then he or she will usually have a blinding headache and not be aware of anyone around them. This is when a need to be quiet and have a sleep takes over. This rest enables the brain to settle back to normal.

I may be classed as ungrateful here, but having well-meaning people hanging over you trying to talk to you asking you your name etc is not good for an epileptic just after having a seizure. You as the victim of epilepsy won't know. Just peace and quiet and a sleep, that is what is needed after an attack. Well it is for me.

* * * * * * * * * *

Section 9

DISADVANTAGES HEALTHWISE

MENUSTRATION... Whenever I menustrated from the age of 13 yrs my seizures increased dramatically over this period then subsided after the cycle finished.

HOSPITALS...On the many, many times when I have been taken to hospital, if I had to stay in for any time then I was always put in a side ward. These side wards were for two reasons that I know of....1 So that if I had an epileptic attack then someone could come to me quickly and 2..So that I would not upset other patients. This even happened when I had my children. Once more I felt like a leper each time I ended up in hospital, and believe me there have been numerous times when this has happened.

INJURIES... I have had quite a few injuries over the sixty odd years; broken collar bones, broken ankle, broken teeth, sprained wrists. All caused by epilepsy. There have been so many I can't remember them all. Banging my head sharply on concrete pavements, knocking myself out; I doubt these helped my epilepsy to get better. These injuries often needed me to be hospitalised overnight.

GLASSES...I have always had to have at least two pairs of glasses, with plastic lenses as I have a few times knocked out the lense when I have had a seizure outside. This has been very expensive over the years.

PREGNANCIES...Throughout each of my four pregnancies my epilepsy was very bad. It was a miracle that at that time I never killed both the children and myself. But they were all healthy children so I was apparently the only one to suffer from the pregnancies.

MARRIAGE...I now firmly believe that marriage is not good for epileptics. Well it was not good for me. The constant stress of relationships and children and home, trying to please everyone, no, it caused me to have more seizures.

INSURANCE...This is one thing I have never been able to obtain...an insurance policy. Insurance companies just will not insure epileptics; they are too big a risk. I have tried all my life to get one but to no avail.

* * * * * * * * * * *

Section 10

SAFETY / ACCIDENTS IN THE HOME

FIRES...A very dangerous subject if you are an epileptic as I have found out to my cost, not in money but health. There are many forms of heating now, much more than when I was young. I will, however, go through the varieties of heating and explain the hidden dangers I have experienced with them.

COAL FIRES...Rarely used now. These can be one of the worst things to live with if you are an epileptic. I had a seizure once and my neighbour found me lying on the tiled grate unconscious after having a seizure. It was related to me later that had I been another two inches and my hair would have been burnt off. That incident frightened me and even before I had the children I always used a large nursery guard around the fire. At least that was one less lethal weapon in the home.

PARAFFIN HEATERS...Definitely not a good form of heating if you suffer from epilepsy. Many years ago I bought a cheap tall black paraffin heater to stand in my kitchen; we never had central heating then! I had a fit in the kitchen and knocked the heater over, lucky for me it was summer, but this made me realise that had it been winter, and had the heater been alight then my whole family would probably have been dead. That went out very quickly to the joy of my father who was a fireman and was always telling me of the dangers of paraffin heaters and fire.

ELECTRIC FIRES....These can be dangerous too, for even with guards they can catch your clothes and skin should you have a seizure and have the bad luck to fall on it. No electric fires for me.

GAS FIRES...I did once have a gas fire for a few years but only when guards were applied to the front. Years ago I had a portable one without any guard and yes, I fell near that and burned my arm so I have never had a gas fire since.

CENTRAL HEATING...Well yes, now we are more advanced regarding heaters and central heating radiators are much safer, I suppose one could still fall on it and burn themselves, but the chances of that happening are very slim I think. When you have had accidents with fires and had a fireman for a father you really do get very wary. I feel safer now with my central heating.

COOKERS...Yes these can cause many of the same problems as fires. Gas cookers are definitely not for Epileptics, one can fall on the gas jet which can in turn blow out the gas flame, the fumes from the cooker can then in turn kill you if you are having a seizure. I had a gas cooker when I first got married but it did not take me long to realise the dangers of these. I then got an Electric cooker. I have always felt much safer with this. Having said that I had a seizure once and burned my arm and wrist slightly. Nothing is that foolproof I suppose when you are an epileptic.

MICROWAVE....I find the microwave oven the safest of all methods for cooking. Plus the added bonus that it turns itself off when cooking is finished. A very good thing if you are, at the time, on the floor having a seizure.

BATHS...Having a bath is not quite as simple for an epileptic. Twice I have nearly drowned because I have had a seizure whilst taking a bath. It is recommended that you only just cover the base of the bath, but that, I do not call a bath. I have had showers installed before moving here, but it has taken me 10 long years to eventually get this council to install a shower for me; I feel much safer now. But all epileptics should have a shower, where possible, it's much safer.

FURNITURE...Another hazard for epileptics. I have twice pulled wardrobes on top of me whilst having a seizure, not at the same time of course. I ended up getting my wardrobes (this was before we had 'built in' wardrobes) fixed to the walls because I have really hurt myself the times that I pulled them on top of me whilst having a seizure. With the Wall Unit in the living room I did the same with that. Once I pulled it on top of me whilst having a seizure, so once more the bolts came out and now it is bolted to the wall. Epileptics are never 100% safe, mainly because with Grand Mal epilepsy the victim never knows when a seizure is going to happen. I know perhaps this sounds rather dramatic but that's what has happened to me; or rather did happen to me.

* * * * * * * * * *

Section 11

IDENTIFICATION

We, as epileptics are always being told by societies that as epileptics we should, as much as possible take responsibility for our own lives and being a sensible person I have always tried to adhere to that idea.

Identity bracelets, we are told are a must and also identification carried on our person. So I got myself a bracelet with my name on and always carry my full name and address in my handbag by way of a diary and notebook. BUT STILL every time I have had a seizure whilst out and have been taken to hospital I have always had ambulance and hospital officials shaking me to ask my name and where I live. Having just come round from a seizure I don't know who I am or where I come from, my blood flow to my brain has not settled down, so however can I be expected to answer these questions.

Not once in over sixty years has anyone ever looked at my bracelet which is very obvious or looked in my bag for my identification. Come on now, I am trying, what about you.

* * * * * * * * * * *

Section 12

HOBBIES AND INTERESTS

SWIMMING...As an Epileptic I have always been very cagey of water and have kept away from Swimming Pools. I've been dragged from a few in the process of having a seizure which is very frightening and eventually I decided to play safe and stay on dry land out of the water.

CAR OWNER...I have always envied people the freedom of having a car, but being an Epileptic I am not allowed a driving licence. It is understandable, I do not wish to kill anyone its just another nail in my coffin so to speak.

DECORATING...Even home decorating, which comes so natural to other people can be a hazard to an epileptic. I like decorating my home but many a time I have had a seizure and fallen off ladders whilst decorating my home. Probably the excitement of seeing the home as you want it. It's a miracle I have not broken my back! I well remember that I once tipped half a tin of emulsion on the carpet.
When I came round, on seeing what had happened I cried for a while but then I cleaned it up and scrubbed it and put another piece of carpet over it. These things can make for a very stressful life if taken too seriously.

HOBBIES...I do try to keep myself fairly busy, doing many things. Writing, knitting, sewing, reading anything so long as it is a challenge. I keep my brain reasonably active. Although now at over sixty years of age I have slowed down. My activities now mainly consist of sitting at the computer writing. If I lived my life wondering when I was going to have another seizure then I would not do anything..ever.

TRAVELLING...I love travelling and have not let my disability stop me. I have travelled by sea, air, train and coach all over the world. Once again I have been very determined not to let epilepsy win. Consequently there have been quite a few accidents on these pursuits I have written about in my autobiography section of this book.

PARTIES AND DRINKING...When I went to parties, (I say this in the past as I don't go out to many now) because I never wanted to be singled out as unsociable I never refused a drink...usually a bit stronger than orange juice I must confess! Unfortunately drink and drugs DO NOT mix. There were however, enough restrictions on my activities in life and so I usually had a lager. The next morning I usually had a bad headache. So I was glad really when my socialising days ended.

MUSIC...This relaxing hobby has been my most rewarding throughout my whole life. Music calms my nerves, providing its not heavy, loud music. Boring as it may sound Easy Listening and Country & Western have been for me the best. Music is like meditation to me. I try to forget everything else. It really does help. Having said that loud music can start my epilepsy off again because I don't like loud music or television so I keep it mellow.

    I often wish that I could start my life again without Epilepsy for there are so many things I have missed out on. Just thinking of all the restrictions to my life though, I suppose I could have ended up with something far worse than epilepsy. I had better be grateful for small mercies even though I still wish I could have been able to have explored life more fully.

* * * * * * * * * *

Part 2

Chapter 1

"SNATCHES OF LIVING"
BY
PEGGY HUME

I was born in 1935, at Woodbridge, in Suffolk. The only child of two working class parents. By the age of five years I had developed Grand Mal Epilepsy, this was diagnosed by the hospital at Ipswich.

My Mum had a hard time looking after me when I was young. She worked part time to pay for my epilepsy treatment; no health service then, and as the 2nd World War was on my Dad was away in the Army. It must have been a worry to her. She had admitted to me that although she always helped me when I had a seizure if she was around, it always upset her seeing me having them even after 64 years of watching me, it still upset her. Probably because she was such a caring person.

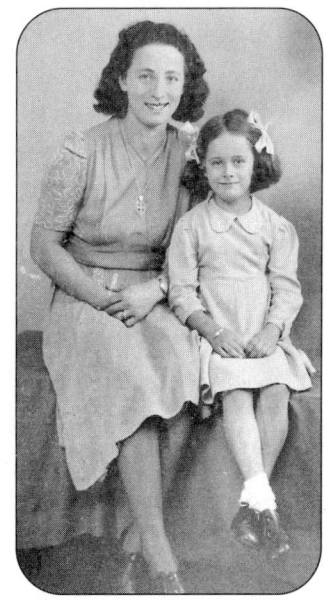

In 1940 when I was first diagnosed as having Epilepsy it was suspected that the Whooping Cough vaccine was to blame, this had been administered when I was a baby. To this day doctors are still not sure if this vaccine contributes to the disease or not with the large amount of people who contract epilepsy in one form or another. I have found that when, I have in the past had a flu injection I have always, around three days later had a seizure. Maybe these vaccines do have something to do with epilepsy. Perhaps more research should be done on this subject.

I can remember clearly my mother and I sitting in this room opposite the consultant in the Neurology clinic at Ipswich Hospital; I was about six at the time so this would have been 1941. He advised my mother to have me put in a home, telling her that I would never get any better, I would be an idiot and no one could help me. Mum sat rigid with her chest out and said "I'm not doing that." The consultant shrugged his shoulders, just muttered something and wrote her out a prescription for the Phenobarbitone to give me daily. Mum guided me out of that room very fast.

My Mum had a hard time of it because I was at that time having an average three Grand Mal seizures daily; she was always being called back from work. She only went to work to pay for the money to get my prescriptions, but she still did it.

Epilepsy in the 1940/50's had not been researched much. There was no technology like we have today in the 2000's. So no one could determine just what was causing the brain disorder. Most people in those days thought, being epileptic we were crazy. Phenobarbitone tablets were about the only known drug to help control the seizures. They never helped me much.

* * * * * * * * * * *

"Snatches of Living"

One of the first things I remember about being an epileptic was when I was attending the Infants School in Woodbridge. It was a small three classroom school. The main entrance was a long red brick hall leading down to the classrooms. It had a brick arch type ceiling and I well remember coming around from the seizures I had daily. I was always laid out in this corridor away from the children on the gym mattress in this long, cold lonely corridor. When I started to come round from the seizure I would lie there praying that someone would come and talk to me, just to remind me who I was and where I was, Eventually I stumbled back into the classroom and the children would giggle. This ridicule hurt me, even then. I spent more time on that mattress than being taught.

I soon realised that I was different from the rest of the children when they were taken out on nature walks. I was never allowed to go with them in case I hurt myself. I was a risk to myself Mum was told; so I would sit alone in the classroom with perhaps one teacher coming and going from the classroom. I would sit there reading until school finished, because my mum was at work.

By the time I went on to the next school at the age of eight when I was trying hard to take in more information the seizures got worse. I seemed to be fighting a losing battle and I was a constant subject of ridicule to the other children. No-one, unless they have been an epileptic can know how this taunting can hurt. I was treated like a leper, someone to be banished to a solitary life. Much of this rejection was instilled in the children, by the parents, who, knowing nothing about epilepsy, treated me as though I had a contagious disease they thought their children could catch. There was little sympathy for me, the epileptic child. No-one understood about epilepsy in the 1930's. We had no television and subjects like epilepsy were not mentioned in the papers or magazines of which there were very few.

* * * * * * * * * * *

Chapter 2

10 YEARS OLD TO TEENS

From the age of five until fifteen years I was having an average three epileptic seizures daily. Often I had only just recovered from one attack when another came on; the constant migraine that accompanied them was something I had to get used to. When I went to sleep I would then have another seizure; called Nocturnal Epilepsy. With these seizures I would find myself juddering around the bed and screaming out in my sleep. By the end of the seizure I had very often fell out of the bed. To solve the problem of falling out of the bed Mum got me a double bed, this helped but I still fell out sometimes if they were very fierce seizures.

* * * * * * * * * *

From the day I was born until I was ten years of age I had spent much of my time with my Great-Grandmother; Dad's Grandmother. She was short lady large in size over twenty stone I expect, with straight white hair. She always wore a crossover pinafore. I can remember only one time when she did not have one on and that was the day she took me up to the post office to open a savings book for me. She was all dressed up smartly, with her coat with a fur collar, a hat and her gloves on, hugging her handbag tightly; I had never seen her look like that. I was quite amazed having never seen it before and I never did again as she became very ill after that and was unable to get out at all. She tucked that savings book in her handbag and said she would see I was alright and we left the post office.

"Snatches of Living"

My Nan owned a sweet shop right opposite the school gates in Woodbridge, because of her deteriorating health, she never left the shop/ home or went outdoors because she had very swollen legs and feet and could not walk far. Had there been the medical tests we have now, then I expect the doctor would have discovered that she had Diabetis, but there were no tests in those days. People just endured illnesses in the 1930's and before, with no known cure. She also had a large goitre probably thyroid deficiency.

Mum always left me with my Nan whilst she went out to work to help with the home/health finances. Nan had a special settee in the living-room for me to lie on when I had my seizures. I would usually be asleep for about two hours but then, once I was conscious I would be offered chocolate toffees; I loved them.

When I was 10 years old, in 1945 the Second World War had just ended. My father returned home from the war to an epileptic daughter who could hardly remember him. Being Epileptic I was a worrier and having this strange man in the house telling me what to do and claiming all Mum's attention was upsetting for me. I was, I suppose a bit jealous of this man turning up out of the blue and changing the life I had lived alone with my mother for nearly six years. Looking back on it I think Dad was jealous of all the attention I was given by Mum when I had seizures and after.

In Jan of 1946; within months of Dad returning home from the war my Nan died. She had been like a second mother to me and now she was gone. I was alone once more in the sense that I spent a lot of time with her when Mum was working and now she was gone forever. I was very upset and missed Nan, this in turn made my epilepsy worse because I worried about it even though I tried to hide it.

By the time I was eleven I left the school I had been attending since eight years old. My epilepsy was no better and the ridicule from the children never helped me. It just continued so Mum moved me to the only other school in Woodbridge; this was affecting my learning because I was upset at the ridicule from the children. This, consequently, was causing even more epileptic seizures.

The situation here was slightly better than the previous school. I tried my hardest to escape the ridicule and rejection by other children, but I rarely did. I tried to prove to them that when I was not 'ON THE FLOOR" as I termed it, I was just as capable as them at learning. I don't think anyone was convinced at that time, although most of the teachers at this second school (The Council School) did seem more sympathetic to my situation.

I must have learned quite a lot though because I passed the eleven plus exams to go to high school. Here however, was another nail in my coffin. There were only four of us girls who passed and the officials refused to let me go because I would have had to travel on a school bus about twelve miles there and back to the high school daily and it was explained that if I had a seizure on the morning bus it would probably effect the other children's learning for the rest of the day. The following year I took the exams once more. I passed again but they refused to let me go on the bus. I just could not win. Mum was getting very angry at all this discrimination against my illness. It seemed I could not win. I daily spent quite a lot of time laid out in the staff room on a settee after having a seizure as I got older. Much more comfortable than those gym mattresses!

I just kept fighting the system; although I never really got anywhere. I was excluded from Cookery classes, Gymnastics classes, Swimming in fact there were very few things I was allowed to attend. I know some of the teachers felt sorry for me; being laid out on yet another gym mattress in the large assembly hall half of the time. No, I never did escape those gym mattresses!

* * * * * * * * * *

The years leading up to my teens were, to say the least, solitary living. A feeling of rejection, a hurtful recognition that you have been made to feel that you are not quite the same as all the other children around you. The most obvious was being treated differently...cautiously would probably be a better word to explain the atmosphere within the school by both teachers and children alike. By fourteen years of age I had become a very introverted young girl.

When I was fourteen my Dad paid for me to have private lessons to learn Shorthand & Typing after being told by a job assessor who had been to the school that it was the only job where I would most probably be safe from injury! I could not work in a factory with machinery. I could not work in a shop with people. Certainly nothing outdoors, so working in an office was the safest answer.

The woman who taught me Shorthand and Typing; Mrs Nesling was her name, was a little woman about 4'9" tall but she really did know about Shorthand. She hated failures and so kept on and on grilling at me until I got it right. Of course at 14 years of age I had other things on my mind!

By now, at school, I was allowed in the Staff Room, not only after a seizure but I did the school filing; I liked filing, seeing everything in correct order, I'm still the same. I also typed their letters and reports up when other children had cookery classes and all the other things which I was not allowed to partake in.

I was by fourteen years of age a reasonably attractive girl and I wanted desperately to impress the opposite sex; boys were on my mind. Also on my mind then was one of the student teachers. His name was Mr Hughes; I really had a crush on him, and I think he liked me. He had jet black hair, was stockily built and about five feet six inches in height. He had wonderful dark brown eyes. I could feel those eyes on me every time we passed each other. I felt elated that he even noticed me. This went on for months until the day I passed out in front of him in the school corridor while we were having a conversation. After that he seemed keen to avoid me. My first experience of how epilepsy can be a killer of romance!

* * * * * * * * * *

Chapter 3

TEENAGE YEARS

By the time I was fourteen, I had started to menustrate, my breasts were filling out and it was obvious that I was on my way to becoming a woman. I could not get there fast enough. My Epileptic seizures had now lessened to an average two daily; one during the day and one during the night. I even had the odd night without one. These did often increase with the menustration period for an average four days until the cycle had finished, then once more the seizures decreased - until the next menustration cycle.

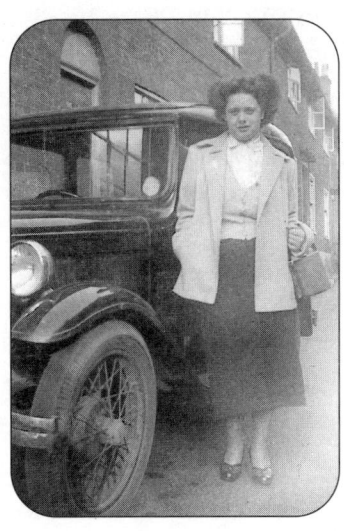

For my 14th birthday Mum took me up to Ipswich shopping for grown up clothes for me. I was so excited. I will never forget that green straight pencil slim skirt which I chose; they were all the fashion that year. It had a slit at the bottom of the back, this made it look very sexy and grown-up. My only thought was: would it impress the boys? To match this Mum bought me a white blouse with a frilled band down the front. To complete the effect, we went to the shoe shop and she got me my first pair of shoes with a heel; only one inch but a heel. I was so excited.

"Snatches of Living"

When we got home I just could not wait to try the outfit on. I looked in the mirror and felt good about myself for about the first time. Here was I, a young girl of fourteen, five feet two inches in height, medium brown curly hair with a minimum amount of make-up; Dad was not keen on make-up and restricted how much I used. People would be surprised when they saw me now and the boys, yes they would probably look too. I wanted them to. Peggy was now not just an epileptic schoolgirl who spent most of her time writhing on the floor having seizures. . At that moment, I was someone to be looked at, not for people to look away from. I felt very good at what I saw in the mirror.

By this time I had acquired one friend who did not let my epilepsy bother her, her name was June, she was nearly the same age as me and lived only six houses away. She never seemed bothered by my epilepsy. If I had a bad attack then she would run for help. If, however it was only a mild one than she would stay with me until I felt well enough for her to walk me home.

Epilepsy can kill romance as I will demonstrate in this incident which I can well remember: I was looking forward to the regular Sunday afternoon walk June and I took around the River Wall in Woodbridge, many boys congregated there; and the girls of course. Boys looking for girls, girls looking for boys. However I will never forget what happened next:

We had all been talking, laughing and generally showing off with the boys for about ten minutes, me in my smart new outfit, looking well-dressed and interesting, the boys naturally watching, when, I was told later I suddenly screamed out and fell to the ground, writhing in the throes of an epileptic seizure. Here I was, one minute becoming a woman and showing myself off, the next second an epileptic shaking and screaming on the ground.

"Snatches of Living"

Probably all revealed underneath! The stunning effect I had hoped for had been tarnished very quickly. I expect, being excited by my new clothes and the effect I hoped they would have on others was what encouraged the seizure.

* * * * * * * * * *

As teenagers we went twice weekly to the Woodbridge Picturehouse. This was, and still is situated in front of the railway station and about once every hour whilst sitting in the cinema, when the train came through the station one could feel the cinema shake. There was an A and B picture on from Monday to Wednesday, and another from Thursday until Saturday evening. Matinee on Saturdays. Very often June and I were sitting there in a picture house full of people, all concentrating when suddenly I would be having a seizure and be screaming and shouting. People would turn and stare. Mr Richardson the cinema manager came and shone his torch, to check if I was all right. June usually waved him away and I would be left in my seat to 'sleep it off' whilst the rest of the audience continued to watch the film. I staggered home after the end of the films, still often in a daze, but June got me there. I was getting much too big to be carried about by anyone. I was just on ten stone in weight with a shapely figure.

At weekends June and I took a chance regarding my having a seizure and went down to Felixstowe, 10 miles away on the bus. We liked going up to Butlins and playing on the juke box there. Us teenagers stood around that machine for hours. I loved music then and still do. Dad never liked me doing this but Mum protested that I had to have some form of life; he gave in but was quick to remind Mum he was right whenever I had a seizure during our outings.

I have spent a large majority of my life in this Jeykll and Hyde existence. Being two completely different people. The epilepsy controlled me and I have struggled continuously to control IT. One of these options could take over at anytime.

* * * * * * * * * *

"Snatches of Living"

Chapter 4

WORK

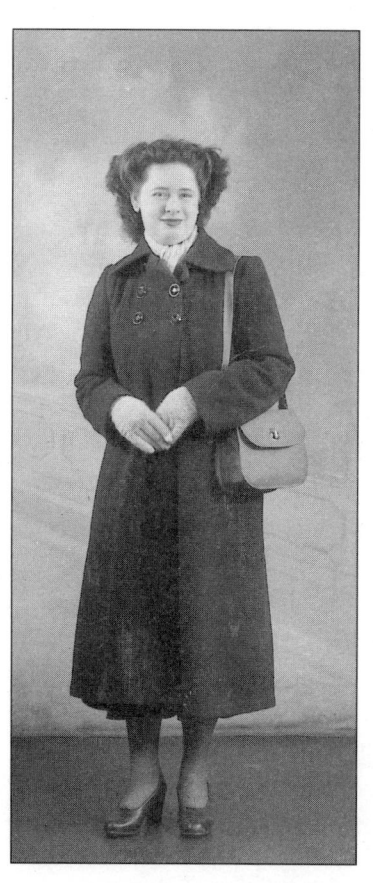

I left school in December of 1950. By then I had accumulated yet another problem: who was going to employ an epileptic who was having a minimum of one seizure everyday? Often during the working hours. There were no such things as help for the disabled. Certainly no Discrimination boards or anything of that sort. If you were refused a job, or were sacked then you just had to accept it. It was hard but that was how it was in those times. I doubt things have changed much now.

I had been advised to get an office job; a sitting down job for safety. I agreed after my experience of office work at school; I quite liked the idea. After much searching, I was eventually offered a job in an office at Ipswich; eight miles from my home. Unless you were a factory worker there were very few jobs in the small country town of Woodbridge where I lived.

Once I acquired this job I travelled on the bus every morning and evening. Need I say that this first job lasted only six weeks due to the employers having had, many times transported me home in cars after I had a seizure at work. On the odd occasion the employers took me to the local hospital until I assured them that, unless I had hurt myself having the seizure, then there was nothing that the hospital could do for me.

From those first few weeks of my working life the ritual was the same at each job: after an average time of two months working. I would be asked in the boss's office and after a lot of apologies and reassurances that it was nothing to do with my work but the epilepsy I would be asked to leave; usually that same day. I was a responsibility which none of them wished to accept. In each incident I was then handed my cards and paid up to the end of the week...some even gave me a little extra money. I suppose its understandable, seeing a person sitting at an interview and passing the tests given and then a few days later seeing that same person writhing and screaming on the floor having a seizure; not quite the same! I was always assured that I could have a reference regarding my capabilities.

In between jobs I spent most days rushing around the Employment Exchanges both at Woodbridge and Ipswich pleading for a job, but the sceptical looks I received when I admitted that I was an epileptic certainly did nothing for my enthusiasm in job hunting.

There were some times when filling out a Job Application form when I got so desperate that, yes I did omit on the form to state that I was an epileptic. That may, to someone who is healthy, sound very deceitful, but desperation is the word I would use. This way I, at least got a chance of proving myself yet again.

* * * * * * * * * *

Yes epilepsy did take over my life. It has been that horrible feeling of inadequacy and the fact that you are different to others. Many times I walked out of the office, after being fired hating myself for who I was and wondering if this, the pattern my life was to go on forever. It did depress me; probably even induced many of the seizures. I certainly was not looking forward to my future life if this pattern was to continue.

The hiring and firing continued so that by the time I was twenty I had been through about twenty jobs. It was so demeaning, this way of life, constantly trying to prove just what I COULD do over what I could NOT do and the worry, well that of course made my epilepsy worse.

In 1968 I had a seizure at work in the office and crushed my right collar-bone on the corner of the office desk. The agonizing pain, I can't think of a word strong enough to describe it. This casualty put me in a coma for a week and hospital for a month. After recovering from this accident; which took two month to heal, I went to the Employment Exchange who, after reading through my health records, advised me that after all the accidents I had had caused by epilepsy that I should apply for a disability pension as the Epilepsy definitely did not seem as if it was going to leave me. I left that office thanking the lady and saying that I would think about it; I was only 33 years old then, I did not want to give up yet, unless I had to. I decided to fight epilepsy a bit longer.

* * * * * * * * * * *

Chapter 5

LATE TEENAGE ROMANCES

From fourteen until sixteen June and I had regular boyfriends we had met in the picturehouse. Mine was over six feet tall, with dark black hair; very attractive too. His name was Bob. June went with his friend, also called Bob. My epilepsy did not seem to distract Bob, we stuck it out for two years and then he joined the Navy and I saw very little of him we spent most of our relationship writing letters. He then met a girl living near his navy base and that as they say was that. I don't think that our parting was solely due to my epilepsy, he just found other attractions.

I was, by this time sixteen years old. June had found a boy she seemed serious about and we went our separate ways, she wanted some privacy and so did I. I then started to go to dances at the Crown Ballroom in Woodbridge on Saturday nights. This was quite interesting as there were a large choice of boys because we had a Royal Airforce base at Martlesham. That was only a mile away. We also had the Americans who were at Bentwaters and other surrounding bases. We really were spoilt for choice.

* * * * * * * * * * *

"Snatches of Living"

EVEN LATER TEENAGE YEARS

I got involved with one of the airmen, doing his National Service at the Martlesham base and after about six months found myself sadly pregnant. Oh dear. In the 1950's women never had the choice of abortions, if she got pregnant she just had to endure the consequences of it and have the baby. That was something shameful to happen. I can't tell you how this upset my dad. He was furious. What was even worse the father of the baby never even wanted to know about my predicament, he disappeared, got another posting to 'escape' his responsibilities once being told by myself and my parents.

My next problem; An epileptic having a baby, how was I going to look after it? I was still having a minimum of two fits daily; one during day and one nocturnal at night. Many questions like this were put to me, both by myself and others. I had no answer. There were no abortion clinics in the 1950's. I must admit it upset me. But, as expected my Dad came back with the answer "YOU PLAYED THE GAME, YOU PAY THE PRICE". I never got any sympathy from him, but I certainly never wanted a child at sixteen years of age. Whatever was I going to do?

* * * * * * * * * * *

I gave birth to a daughter in Feb of 1954, just after my 17th birthday. It was a natural birth; just on four hours in labour. After giving birth my daughter was put in my arms for about five minutes and then I saw the nurses whispering and she was immediately snatched from my arms and taken from me. The sister explained to the nurses that, as had been decided by my parents, (I went along with the idea because I had no choice) she was to be fostered and therefore I was to have no contact with her whilst I was in hospital. I was reminded that I was epileptic and I might drop her anyway. Not a very good excuse.

Over the next five days whilst in hospital I pined for my daughter. Watching when all the other mothers had their babies with them at feeding times. The hospital staff came and advised me to express my breast milk so as to give my daughter a better start in life.

I went many times and stood outside the nursery, hoping to get a chance to hold her just for a few minutes but that chance never came. I spent many sleepless nights crying for my daughter who had been taken from me. I left that hospital feeling so alone; as if part of me was lost completely. Dad picked me up in the car and not a word was mentioned about my daughter I had given birth to; I don't think he even asked me how I was. It was as if she did not exist. Unless you have experienced it personally no-one could understand the torment I felt at having to leave my baby in that hospital. I was told that I deserved it by Dad when I cried once home with them, but no-one deserves the torment of having to give away a child to whom they have just given birth; not knowing where your new-born baby is going. Not unless the mother wants it that way.

Even though my daughter had been taken from me, or as it was put to me 'I gave her up' I never ever forgot her even after having other children. I thought of her every year and wondered as the years went on how she was and how her life had progressed. There would always be that part of me which was missing.

I did meet up with my daughter when in my fifties. We got on reasonably well but not well enough to accept that we were mother and daughter. Our meetings, of which there were a few, deteriorated and its now been over seven years since we met up. It was just not meant to be, there were too many years left between us and other people involved. Our lives, it seems are not compatible now.

* * * * * * * * * *

Chapter 6

MARRIAGE AND CHILDREN

In 1955, eighteen months after my giving birth to my illegitimate daughter, at the age of 19 years I met my future husband, he was a year older than I. An Irishman and a real charmer. He was 5ft 2inches in height, I am 5ft 1inch which made us quite compatible. He was a reasonably nice looking man with a mass of red-brown hair and I adored him. It seemed as though there was nothing that would keep us apart; even epilepsy.

We courted for roughly two months and decided that we both wanted to marry each other. By this time he had seen me have about three seizures whilst in his company. He was adamant that they never worried him, but I was not totally convinced. I evaded the fact that I was an epileptic when I was with him.

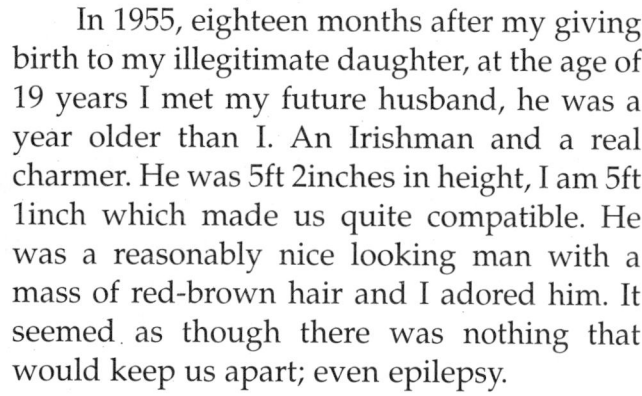

My father and mother tried hard to dissuade him against our marriage, explaining all the responsibilities of living with an epileptic entails. He, however, was not going to be put off, and so two months from the time of meeting we married in Woodbridge church. A very simple wedding without any trimmings.

Dad would not let me wear white because I had given birth to an illegitimate child eighteen months before so I was not a virgin; I think, indirectly, this was his punishment to me for my having had my illegitimate daughter in my teens.

It was a very quiet wedding. I was scared that I would have a seizure but I didn't. There were not very many people invited; just a few family. Not my husband's family as they lived in Belfast. Yes, a very quiet wedding. We rented a bedsit in a large house at Ipswich and after the wedding we just got on the bus, held hands and went to our bedsit in Ipswich. But at that time it did not matter, we were very happy, and in love, I thought.

I continued to work in Ipswich but it did not last long, once more I got my cards; within six weeks of marriage. I suppose married life was already getting to me. I had only been married for six weeks when I got my first black eye. His hobby was boxing for the R.A.F. but I think he was practising on me most of the time. Each time after hitting me he said he was sorry and it would never happen again, many times he cried and I naturally believed him, but it always did happen again. I doubt these beatings helped my epilepsy, the constant bangs which he gave me to my head when he hit me probably make the epilepsy worse. Not to mention the stress and tension I endured from the beatings, it was terrible. He kept on cruelly reminding me for the next seven years that I was lucky he married me and no-one else would have married an epileptic. That hurt, I could not help being epileptic. It certainly was not an illness I chose to have.

Within two months of marriage I was pregnant, we never had The Pill or other contraceptive methods in the 1950's, only the condom and a lot of men did not like wearing them, my husband included. Now I had no job, was pregnant and had a husband who regularly knocked me about. He spent the money as it came in on drink and gambling. Never considering the household bills and rent, the children and who was going to pay for them? He was always stealing from my purse. What had I got myself into?

* * * * * * * * * *

"Snatches of Living"

Mum found us a little cottage in Woodbridge, practically back-to-back to where she lived. It only took us five minutes to get to each other's home. The cottage had a kitchen, a front room, a small sitting room and two bedrooms. We had only the toilet up the top of the garden and a bathroom was a luxury we never had in 1950's. The house and three others side by side were privately owned by a man living near. We paid the landlord five shillings a week rent, an average weekly rent then.

We could have been very happy if my husband had curbed the drink/ women and rash spending. But he never gave anything to the marriage, never had any money and never gave a thought about what I, or the children needed. He never, ever took me out.

Within five years I had given birth to three children. With each pregnancy I spent a minimum of eight hours of every sixteen daylight hours having, and recovering from epileptic seizures. I got terrible attacks of migraine after the seizures. Luckily the children slept well when little, I understand now that it was probably something to do with the drugs I was taking for epilepsy, which after my breast-feeding got in the babies system, consequently they slept more.

My doctor increased the dosage of Phenobarbitone through each of my pregnancies. I felt like a zombie. I just wanted to sit down or sleep all the time. I could not concentrate on a book for many minutes and I have always loved reading books, it was a terrible way of living; an existence. But as any woman knows, once you have a crying baby then it is impossible to sleep or have any quiet moments to yourself for long even when you have a splitting headache. Plus being drugged to slow down my brain never helped the situation.

I don't think anyone in my family; least of all my husband, had any idea how these high doses of medication for epilepsy affected me as a person. I tried very hard to snatch moments of living for myself but it never lasted. Sympathy I never got. I was told I just had to live with my mistakes; and I did.

After the birth of my youngest son Paul, I was advised to have a sterilization whilst I was still in hospital after his birth. I was told it was for the good of my health and would probably stop me having so many seizures. I certainly was not living life to the full at this time and even sterilization would be worth it if the seizures were less. My husband did not seem to care; he was rarely there now. He was always getting postings away from home. Our marriage was ended anyway.

Throughout our seven year marriage I was so traumatized by living the way I was that I got to the stage where I tried to kill myself at least twice whilst being married to my husband, it never worked and I was told by the hospital staff that trying to kill myself would probably never work because my body was so used to the tablets that an overdose would not be effective. What was I going to do?

After the sterilization operation I was no longer worried about getting pregnant; it has a 90% success rate. That was one problem hopefully removed. So when my husband did come home, which was very rare I, at least did not have to worry about another pregnancy if intercourse did happen..

Finally, after seven years of violence/two nervous breakdowns where I spent long periods in a nursing home/two suicide attempts/three children and six wasted years I decided this was no life for an epileptic, so I took action. I got a legal seperation from my husband in 1959, he was hardly ever at home with us now so it was not going to really be any different; just legal and it would stop him hitting me constantly. My turmoil was about to lessen, if I had my way. I was determined about that.

* * * * * * * * * * *

Two years later, my husband came to the house with the excuse of seeing the children. Sadly I did not hear the warning bells once again. I had been alone with three children for over a year and was glad of male company; even my ex husband.

The last eighteen months living alone with the three children had helped my epilepsy. The seizures had definitely decreased without the worries of finance and emotional problems which having a husband had brought me. I could sometimes go without one a whole day and just have the nocturnal ones so I felt better; not for long.

My husband had a posting to R.A.F Singapore and pleaded, that day he visited me, for me and the children to go for a year with him. I gave in eventually and he went out there and we followed on a few weeks later. I gave up my home and that was that. Well I really should have known better, knowing my husband.

We had only been out there about two weeks when he started coming home late from work; eleven in the evening instead of five. Drunk as usual. He was going around with other women, our Armah included. He was never going to change.

After just over three months of being back with him his playing around with women, me having endured endless seizures, his nearly killing me and my ending up in hospital time after time through his cruelty to me, and the kids staying with neighbours for two weeks. It was arranged by the R.A.F. for myself and the three children to come back to England in a hospital comet, three days before Christmas 1962.

* * * * * * * * * * *

"Snatches of Living"

On arriving back in England from Singapore; with two large black eyes and bruises all over I had no idea where we were to go, apart from visiting my parents. I had no home for myself and three children. Barely any furniture; apart from a few stored items. We would need a three-bedroom house now with the children getting older. The council had nothing to offer us. And there were no 'safe-homes' in the 1960's for abused families. This worry started off my epilepsy very bad, two seizures a day again.

I obtained a divorce on Cruelty and that was the last time I ever saw him.

* * * * * * * * * *

Chapter 7

WHERE IS HOME?

After our return to England talking many days with my parents (who had only a two bedroom house) it was finally decided that until I could get an allocation of a council house I was to take a housekeepers job. I was quite a good cook and I would leave the two eldest children; nearly six and four with my parents and take Paul my 2-year old with me. I took a job as a housekeeper about sixteen miles from Woodbridge. I just made sure that the man knew I was epileptic but he agreed to give it a trial and I went.

* * * * * * * * * *

I kept pressing the local council but it was five years 1966 before I was offered a council house in Woodbridge. My children had been spoiled by my parents in that time and now did not want to leave them. I could not afford the rent of a three-bedroomed house just for myself and my son Paul so I took a dingy bedsit in Felixstowe where I could be alone with my son. It was not a very nice place but my husband never, ever, paid the maintenance as the courts had ordered; he kept changing addresses so as not to be found.

The epilepsy eased a bit and I took on part-time jobs. During the day in an office and the odd evenings as a bar maid, to help with the mounting bills and finances. This way of life, an existence I would call it, went on for about a year and then my son Paul died of stomach cancer . He was buried on his birthday in December, 1967. Whatever was happening to my life? Was there no end to the problems.

I summed my life up. I now had no children with me, no home of my own, no job, in fact nothing to look forward to at all. What was I going to do next I asked myself. Plus I was still having epileptic seizures, although many days I got away with having just the one seizure at night.

I had no relationships with any men to this time. All the terrible worries of relationships from the past made me realise that marriage and family life was not for me, at least not with a man who knocked me about constantly. It would take two to work together for it to work properly and he was too immature for that.

* * * * * * * * * *

Chapter 8

PLANNING THE REST OF MY LIFE

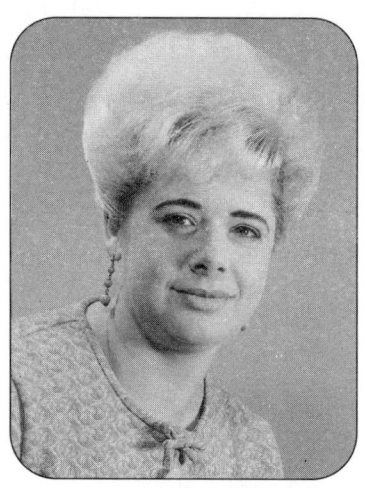

TRAVELLING

After another year; to 1968, I was feeling an intense loneliness. I now had no children with me, although I did go to see them every week. I tried many times to claim back my children from my parents but was reminded each time that the children staying with them was for their good. Reminding me that I was an epileptic, as if I had a contagious disease. I should have listened to my own head instead of letting others make the decisions for me regarding my children, but I can't turn the clock back. I felt at the time it was for their good and I gave in.

It was useless worrying about the situation regarding the children, they just did not want to leave my parents. If I worried about the situation it only induced more seizures and then I could not work or do anything. I had to plan something to do with my life.

* * * * * * * * * *

It was a few months after Paul my son died and I was working my evening shift in the pub when I got talking to a young man. He called himself Peter and said he was a rep from London. He sat for about three hours telling me what a wonderful place London was and that I should go. He assured me that as I had a bubbly personality I would mix well with people. He also assured me that I would have no trouble getting work there. I was intrigued, it certainly sounded interesting. I thought about this idea and within two weeks I had packed my bags and left for London. I was 33 yrs at this time. Where in London I was going I did not know. I never realised what a large place it was. But he was right there were opportunities if you knew where to look.

I rented a bedsit upstairs in a house in Ealing. It was nice and clean. The people seemed very friendly. Once in the room I stood my cases down and just laid on the bed staring at the ceiling, what had I let myself in for now? How had I, a country girl ended up here in London? The tears fell down the sides of my face. I assured myself that I had to calm down to avoid the epileptic seizures returning in large amounts!

I spent the next few days looking for a job and got one as a telex operator in Tottenham Court Road in London. It lasted about three months and once more the hiring and firing started again, and the epilepsy naturally also got worse again with the worry between jobs.

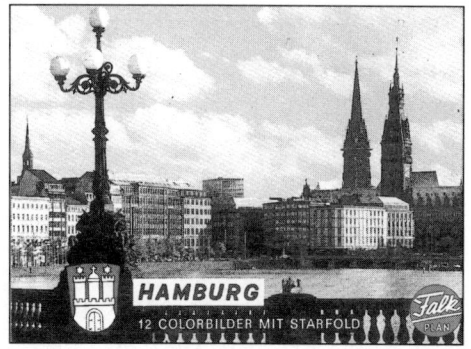 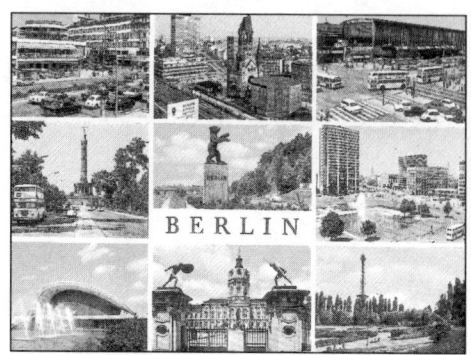

This way of life went on for nearly four years, with numerous seizures between jobs but then my luck changed and I was offered a job in Hamburg with the sister company of the shipping company I was working for in London to work for them in Hamburg, Germany. I was given three months to learn the basics of German language and I was away.

I have always loved travel and the flight never worried me at all. I just prayed that I did not greet them with a seizure! I worked for the shipping company in Hamburg for just on a year. I still had the odd seizure but I stuck it out; I was enjoying myself between seizures!

* * * * * * * * * * *

"Snatches of Living"

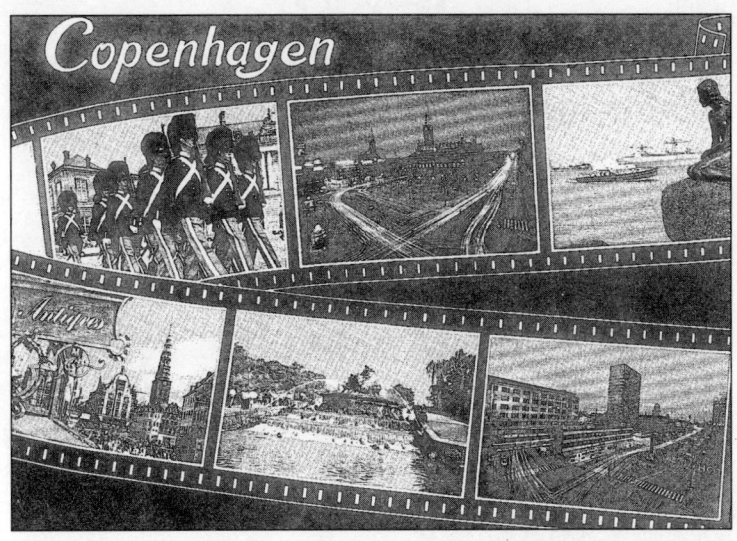

During the time working in Hamburg I got friendly with a girl Margaret also from England. Every alternate weekend we took off to places like Sweden, Holland, Amsterdam, Berlin the list was endless. Germany is a central point, so it is easy to get to all these places. We stayed in hostels all over and if I had a seizure Margaret just sat me down (just as June had done earlier in my life) until I was ready to move on. But I never gave up and we really did enjoy life. I was lucky to have a friend like Margaret, who, by her tolerance made my travel life possible. After the years contract I returned to London.

* * * * * * * * * *

Chapter 9

CAIRO

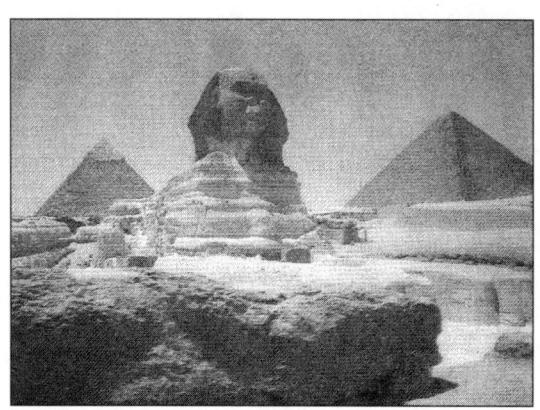

Thinking back I suppose about the most dramatic event concerning these epileptic seizures was after returning to England. I got an Egyptian boy friend and we were getting very serious. He asked me to go to Cairo, Egypt to meet his parents and stay for a while; the time was left unlimited.

Without another thought I booked the next flight, put my possessions in storage and I got a direct flight to Cairo. Whilst on the flight I had a very bad seizure, the crew were so worried because they could not revive me that they re-directed the flight to Beiruit Airport and took me to the Beiruit Hospital. I was made to stay overnight and after a check-up the next morning was put on the next flight to Cairo; I was a day late but after all the excitement I got there! As my boy-friend had not seen me have a seizure I made the excuse that another passenger had been taken ill. More evasive actions to evade telling the truth about epilepsy.

I was caught up in Cairo in the 1973 October war and was not allowed out of the country. However after a few days the officials changed their mind and sent all foreign visitors back to their countries, wherever. The only trouble here was we had to pay for our own flights etc. It was decided that the people who had no money would then get the bill when back in their own home country. More problems.

* * * * * * * * * *

"Snatches of Living"

Chapter 10

BACK HOME IN ENGLAND

I arrived back in England about a week later after train and boat journeys from Cairo. I was on the night train about 3-4 days, it's a long while ago now. Here I was back in London again. I was lucky enough to get the same bed-sitter I had had previously. The epilepsy; with all these troubles was getting very bad now, at least two seizures a day and another in the night. Back to the stress and old health problem - Epilepsy.

I took on a few more jobs, but nothing permanent. I then remembered what the woman at the Employment Exchange had advised me regarding getting a Disability Pension and being registered disabled. I was never going to be able to hold a job permanently. I gave in regarding the disability pension. After a medical examination it was agreed that I was not capable of working and a few weeks later I was sent an invalidity pension book.

After literally being stamped as Registered Disabled, not a pleasant thing, but I felt in a sense relieved that I no more had to fight the system but at the same time I felt totally useless. It is very demeaning to come to terms with the fact that you are of no use to anyone. Well that's how they see you. I did, on the other hand, realise that I would not have all the stress of early mornings and travel daily; some of the things which had certainly made my epilepsy worse. Perhaps the seizures would lessen now. Hopefully, I could only try to help myself, whether it would work I was not sure.

WHAT NOW?

I now felt that I had to do something with my life. Sitting at home doing nothing all day made me feel very unsettled. I have a very active brain. I decided to learn something and so I went to the City of Literary Art, Drury Lane, London where it was possible, and still is to learn anything. I decided to take up Writing and Psychology classes (people's brains and the way they think fascinated me). I then saw, and other tutors saw that even though I was an Epileptic I had some talents. I stayed in London for another three years, studying, writing, pushing myself as far as I dare and enjoying my chosen subjects. But I did eventually have a yearning for East Anglia and my family again.

* * * * * * * * * * *

It was now 1976, my epileptic seizures had lessened; sometimes I went two or three days in between seizures; obviously a quieter life suited me. I now had a council flat in Hayes, Middlesex.

Just looking through the exchange list whilst in the council offices one day I noticed there was an exchange for Saxmundham, only 12 miles from my home in Woodbridge. I phoned the man up who had been given a job in London. He lived in a bungalow and was desperate to get to London and I wanted to come home and so we had a mutual exchange within the week. That was May, 1976. Soon I would be back home. Nearly back where I had started from. I would see my family more now. It felt good.

* * * * * * * * * * *

Chapter 11

A TRUE FRIEND

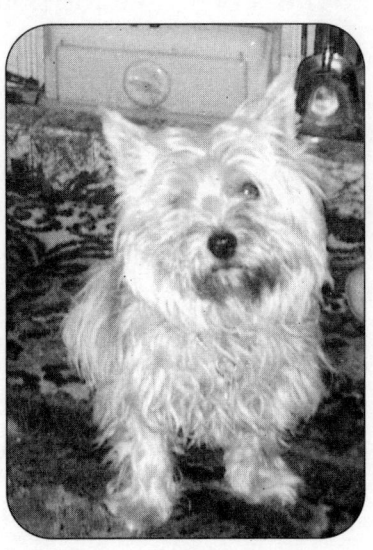

After a few months I felt a bit lonely. Living in the country is not the same as living amongst the hustle and bustle of London. The country life is a much more solitary, quieter way of life.

Now I had so much time on my hands I decided to get myself a dog. I got a Cairn puppy dog. I called him Whisky. He was beige in colour; a wheaten. I was later to find that he was my best friend.

Whenever I had an epileptic seizure he came and laid on my chest until I started coming round where he could see my eyes moving. He would then lick my face to bring me round; like an indoor private doctor! He watched my every movement for hours after the attack.

He never seemed at all frightened, as some humans, in fact he seemed to like to mother me; like it was his job and he was only doing it. We looked after each other.

I well remember two incidents where he saved my life whilst I was having an epileptic seizure. Had it not been for his thinking, (they must have brains) I would have died. The first happened when he was about three years old. I was having a bath and always left the bathroom door ajar or he would bark at the door, he wanted to check on me all the time. I could not have been in the bath many minutes when I had a seizure. Whisky, the dog must have immediately jumped in the bath on his rescue mission and within a few minutes I could feel him lightly scratching at my neck and pawing my face. His actions awoke me and when I was aware of what had happened I got out of the bath and went to lie on the bed...the dog following behind me.

I was lucky that time I was saved by two factors: I had a very short bath so I had not slid completely under the water and the dog clawing tenderly at my face had revived me. That incident frightened me and from then I got myself a shower extension. Just how close had I come to the end?

The second incident happened one winters' day. It was cold and I decided to have sausage and chips for dinner to warm me up. The sausages were sizzling in the frying pan and the chips were in the chip pan when I suddenly had a seizure. I was lying on the floor unconscious for what must have been quite a while. It was revealed to me later by neighbours what next took place, as I myself was oblivious to anything.

When cooking I always left a tiny kitchen window open. A person going past had seen streams of smoke coming from my kitchen window. I lived in a cul-de-sac where the kitchen was visible from the road. The dog was apparently barking frantically. By this time the kitchen was a ball of flames.

The man called the fire brigade immediately and when they arrived the poor dog had practically passed out himself from smoke inhalation.

Both the dog and myself were dragged out onto the grass verge outside my kitchen door to recover and the fire was put out. When I came round later I saw this black smoke still billowing from the kitchen. I stumbled into the kitchen only to see a mass of black walls and smoke. A sorrowful sight which I shall never forget and poor Whisky the dog, staggering in there behind me. A neighbour had come in behind me and lain me on the bed after the seizure and the dog stayed with me.

Later when I awoke from the sleep and stumbled into the kitchen, I burst into tears. All this damage caused by me having an Epileptic seizure. It was also revealed to me when the neighbour came into check on me later that it had been the dogs loud barking and strange noises which had drawn the man's attention to the flames. So once more Whisky saved my life.

Those two incidents alone show how vulnerable an epileptic is to death if things go wrong. In that situation the chip pan had caught fire and splashed fat around the frying pan and the lighted electric plate and whoosh! That's how easy it can happen.

I had Whisky the dog for fifteen years and then he contracted bowel cancer, he was a sorry sight because he hated his 'accidents' indoors and the vets advised me that he was in pain and to have him put to sleep. I eventually gave in but oh, how I miss him. He looked after me as an epileptic for years. I felt safe whilst I had him. Now I had nothing and no-one again, I had to look after myself once more. I would never find another dog like him. I live in a flat now and dogs are not allowed so I just stare at his photograph and remember. I have a lot of years of caring to thank him for.

* * * * * * * * * * *

"Snatches of Living"

SUMMARY OF LIFE

Even though I had an 'affliction/brain disorder' call it what you will, (I have certainly called it some very nasty names throughout my life), I have fought with it all my life. I have done many of the things I wanted to do. There are a few I was not allowed to do. I travelled, I did many things I was told were not possible for an epileptic. I never gave up. My only real regret was not being allowed to drive a car. I would have loved that luxury, the freedom; a wonderful thought. Much better than public transport. Being epileptic one just has to be sensible and know where to draw the line. You could kill yourself. Epilepsy is so unpredictable, or it might never happen again. Who can tell, we can't.

Now due to advances in medicines for epilepsy my health has improved, I don't know if age has anything to do with it. I can often go three months or more without a seizure which makes life much easier. This does not mean that the Petit Mal has gone completely. I often get strange feelings and then I know it is time to lie down for a while, a sort of warning signal. I have to live with them…I don't have any option do I?

The deterioration of the seizures is probably due to a very much less hectic life-style, with less aggravation and worry. I must say however, that when I do have the seizures now they take much longer to get over. Its apparently to do with the deterioration of brain cells as we get older. So a seizure which twenty years ago would have taken me two HOURS to recover from can now take me two DAYS to recover from. That problem makes hard going sometimes, I often feel very angry that two days of my life are once more missing.

My only fear is that I will, at my age of over 60 years have a stroke whilst having a seizure. This is my most scary thought. I know it is possible. I just hope it never happens.

I do a lot of writing now. Writing this has made me come to terms with epilepsy, even if I can't control it completely. That does not mean that I don't still hate it. I do, but as they say "You have to live with it."

Advantages of being an epileptic? No I cannot say there have been any. I live with it because I have no choice, but it will *NEVER* be my friend.

* * * * * * * * * * *